THE FADING GARDEN:
A DAUGHTER'S JOURNEY WITH DEMENTIA

by Gail S. Turner-Day

Dedication

To My Dearest Mother, Nancy Turner,

You were the radiant bloom in the garden of our lives, a fragile yet enduring flower that brought beauty and love to every season. Your presence, though dimmed by the relentless passage of time, has left an indelible mark on our hearts. As I stand amidst the fading petals of memory, I dedicate these words to you, my guiding light.

To My Family,

You stood by my side, each of you, a resilient stem in the garden of our collective strength. Together, we weathered the storms that dementia brought into our lives. Through every wilting moment, we found solace in one another's support, nurturing the memories we held dear, and watering the bonds that make us who we are.

To My Friends,

You were the raindrops that refreshed my soul when I needed it most. Your unwavering friendship provided the sustenance to withstand the challenges of the dementia journey. In your understanding smiles and comforting words, I found the strength to keep moving forward.

In the garden of life, we learned that even as the colors fade, and the blooms wilt, the essence of love remains evergreen. My mother, Nancy, may have embarked on her final journey through the twilight of dementia, but her love and legacy will forever flourish in our hearts.

As the garden of memory continues to fade, we will cherish the moments we shared, tending to the delicate petals of remembrance. In the stillness of the garden, we find solace, knowing that love transcends time and memory.

With warmth and heartfelt gratitude,

Gail

TABLE OF CONTENTS

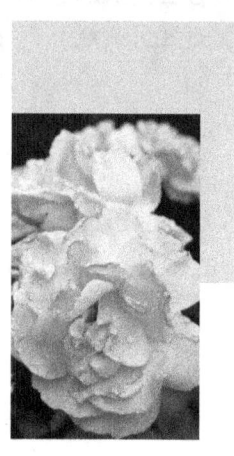

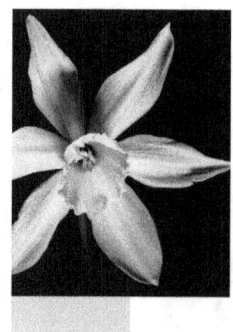

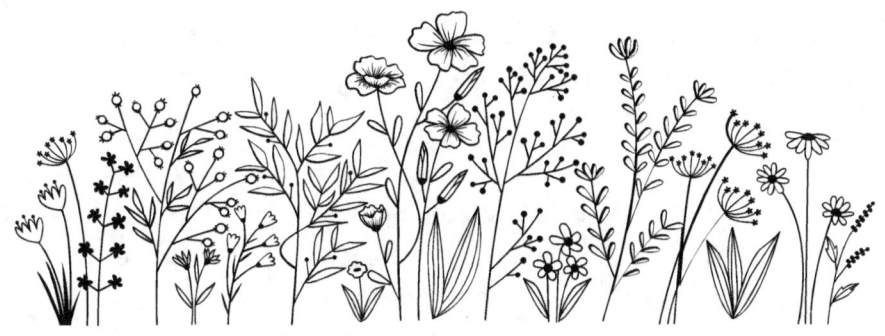

PURPOSE AND FORMAT

This book is all about helping you navigate the challenging journey of dementia, whether you are caring for a loved one or facing an early diagnosis yourself. I learned from my experience that my journey was disjointed, with unknown twists and turns, no guidepost for me to follow so I have taken a thoughtful and structured approach to address the often confusing and unpredictable nature of this journey. My main goal is to be your guiding light, offering support and insights every step of the way.

Reflection Pages: These special pages are like a quiet moment for your thoughts and feelings, and you will find one in each chapter. They are here to help you think things through and understand your emotions better. Using these pages is important because they can improve your mental health during this tough journey.

Coping Skill Exercises: In this book, you will come across some helpful exercises to cope with the tough times. Think of them as small but effective tools and tips, inspired by what I used to cope. They are here to lend you a hand in handling the everyday ups and downs of anxiety and frustration. These exercises are like a shield for your emotions, keeping you strong and preventing those moments when emotions might overwhelm you or make you want to step back from your loved ones.

Affirmation Pages: Inside these parts of the book, you will find words that lift your spirits. They are like little boosts of hope and positivity. These words are here to help you swap out those bothersome negative thoughts with brighter ones, giving your emotional well-being a nice lift.

Resource Repository: And finally, I wanted to include resources you could access that will provide you with more information to help you understand what is happening to your loved one. By the time my mother was in the late stage, I did not have the energy to "do research."

This book will help you get started.

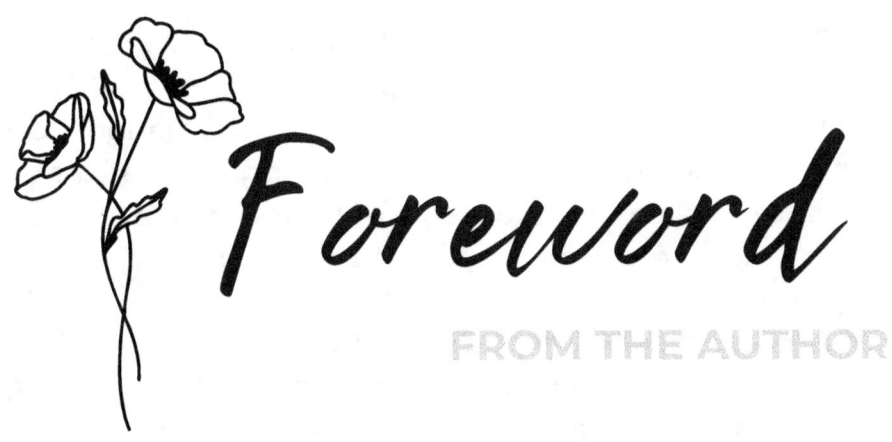

Foreword

The Garden: The Process of Dementia

She laid peacefully in her hospital bed, with a glow of calm, peace and release, holding my hand asking, "You know I love you". And my response, with tears in my eyes was "Yes, and you know I love you too." She took her last breath with dignity at 99.

It can be difficult to describe the experience of a loved one transitioning into dementia, as the journey can be complex and different for each person. However, one way to think about it is to imagine a beautiful garden that gradually becomes overgrown and tangled as time goes on.

The seasons change and as time passes, the garden begins to show signs of neglect. Weeds start to grow, the soil becomes dry, and the flowers begin to wilt.

As the garden continues to be neglected, it becomes harder to distinguish the individual plants and flowers from one another. The once clear paths and walkways become overgrown and tangled, making it difficult to navigate the garden.

In a similar way, a loved one with dementia may gradually become less able to navigate the complexities of daily life. They may struggle to remember important information, lose track of time, and have difficulty completing familiar tasks. Over time, the once vibrant aspects of their personality may become harder to recognize as their condition progresses.

Dementia is a group of symptoms that are associated with a decline in cognitive function, including memory loss, difficulty with language, disorientation, and changes in mood and behavior. Dementia can be caused by a variety of factors, including Alzheimer's disease, brain injury, and vascular diseases.

According to recent statistics, women are disproportionately affected by dementia. Approximately two-thirds of people with dementia are women, and women are also more likely to be caregivers for those with the disease. The reasons for this disparity are not entirely clear, but some factors that may contribute include a longer life expectancy for women and a greater likelihood of women experiencing risk factors for dementia, such as stroke and hypertension.

The purpose of my story is to provide some personal insight on the struggles I faced during this unknown journey and provide information as a resource. Do I have all the answers to all the questions? No, but it is a light on the road to know what lies ahead, knowing where the curves are, the bumps, the speed limits, the areas of caution, the speed traps, and the estimated time of arrival, like the GPS.

REFLECTIONS

Take time to read and process the question before writing. The purpose of this exercise is to allow you to get in touch with your thoughts and emotions. By writing them down, you gain an understanding of our thoughts and feelings more clearly.

What feelings, thoughts, or emotions are emerging from reading the previous passage?

My Strength is Greater Than any Struggle

WAYS TO COPE

Think of coping skills as tools in your mental toolbox to help you better understand and manage your emotions. These are your lifelines when anxiety tries to pull you under. In the pages ahead, we will explore a variety of coping skills, each designed to address various aspects of anxiety.

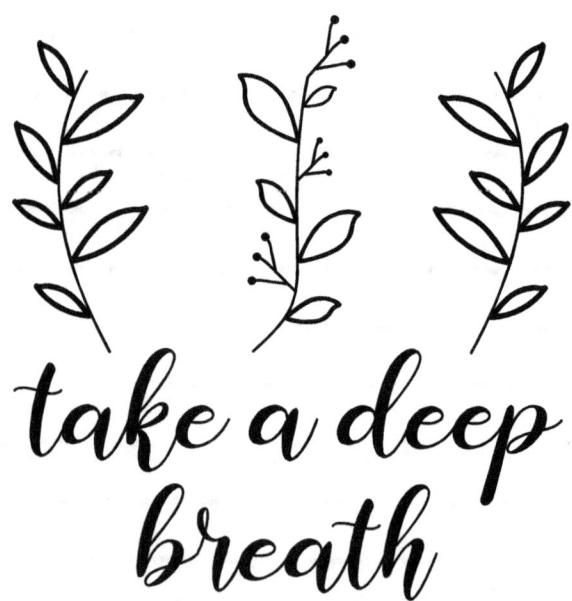

take a deep breath

Practice deep breathing. Inhale deeply through your nose for a count of **four**, hold for **four**, then exhale slowly through your mouth for a count of **six**, repeating as needed until you begin to feel lighter.

10 Daily Affirmations For Alzheimer's and Dementia Caregivers

1. I am doing the best I can do. I should not fear what tomorrow holds, but take each day as a chance to learn something new and grow my confidence as a caregiver.

2. When I am frustrated, I will take a few deep breaths and remind myself that patience is a virtue I can and will embrace.

3. I need to take care of myself to be here tomorrow. Is there something I am neglecting to do for my own health and well-being?

4. Worry is my worst enemy. I am in control of my thoughts and should focus on what I can control, and accept things I can't change.

5. If it were me being cared for, I would want my caregiver to (fill in the blank).

6. The energy I bring to each day has power. It is up to me to make it positive and joyful.

7. I am thankful for this day and the chance to live, love, and provide care to someone who needs me.

8. I will reach out to others if I need a helping hand today from a friend or family member.

9. When it's time to rest, I will rest! Sleep is an essential necessity I should never ignore.

10. I need to give myself credit for what I do every day. It takes a very strong person to do what I do and I am proud of myself.

TotalHomeCareSupplies.com | Caregiver Corner

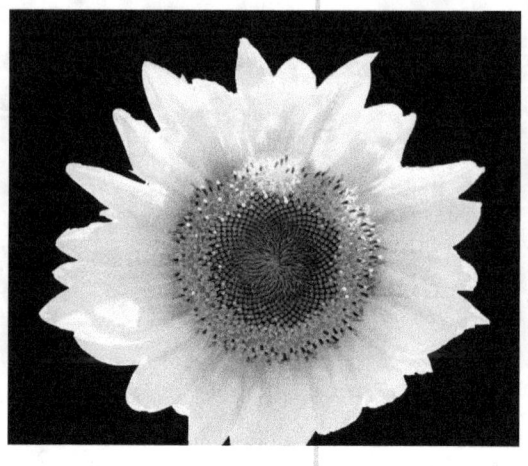

Early memories - The Good Times

A vibrant figure in the tapestry of our lives, my mother was affectionately known as "Sweet Nancy." Her presence radiated warmth, and her infectious humor endeared her to everyone she met. But it was her knack for seamless management that truly stood out. A true taskmaster, she orchestrated her world with meticulous precision. Call it an obsession, but she maintained a comprehensive ledger of every interaction, every conversation, all neatly documented. The billing discrepancies? They did not stand a chance. A 99% success rate of rectification showcased her formidable determination.

Then there were her legendary pound cakes. With the memory of a seasoned baker, she whipped up those iconic creations, churning them out like clockwork on an imaginary cake production line. Pound cakes were her gifts, her tokens of affection for every occasion. From hospital visits to church gatherings, nursing homes to birthdays, and celebrations to simple expressions of love, her pound cakes were omnipresent.

She had honed her skills to such an extent that she could even freeze them! A seemingly audacious feat that defied conventional baking wisdom.

However, time has a way of reshaping even the most cherished narratives. As she reached her 90s, the reliable cadence of her cakes began to falter. The once perfect memory recipe began to slip away, and her mental notes took the place of a once flawless symphony. The bakery of cherished memories gradually gave way, the rhythm slowing as dementia's grip began to tighten.

A true social butterfly, my mother thrived in the company of others. Card games were her chosen arena, and she relished every moment spent playing. She even claimed the title of the "Straight Whist Queen." Hours would vanish as she remained absorbed in her chosen pastime. But, like the shifting tides of an ever-changing sea, her interest in family gatherings underwent a transformation. The absence of her presence during Thanksgiving, Christmas, and Easter dinners was like a ripple through our hearts.

Then came March of 2020, a fateful month that claimed my brother due to COVID-19. He had been a co-caretaker in the journey through dementia with my mother. A year earlier, my father had also passed away due to heart failure. He had witnessed the progression of my mother's dementia through its various stages. His tales of her erratic behavior, sundowning, restlessness, and even violent outbursts painted a picture of a person I did not recognize. The empathy and compassion that once defined her, seemed to have evaporated.

Visits to my parents' home transformed into scenes of quietude, with my father retreating into a corner while my mother's behavior escalated. Tantrums erupted, kitchen counters bore the brunt of her frustration, and I struggled to comprehend the transformation. She was becoming a stranger, and the emotions that swirled around her were a tempest within me.

Through all this, one irrefutable truth emerged: something was wrong. Slowly but surely, the pieces of the puzzle fell into place. I began to suspect that my mother's behavior was not merely a result of mood swings or stubbornness. The realization that dementia might be at play began to dawn on me.

As her Primary Care Doctor shed light on her behaviors, the connection to dementia became undeniable. This marked the initiation of a new phase in our lives, a journey into the intricate maze of dementia. It was a realm unfamiliar to me and my immediate family, a territory we had never navigated before. The shifts were seismic, and we were just beginning to grasp the significance.

Life is filled with Post-it Notes...
Organizing & Compartmentalizing...

BUT GOD

IS THE NOW!

One word, one direction, one focus...

HIM

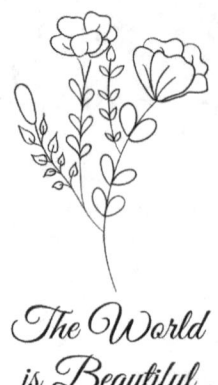

The World is Beautiful

REFLECTIONS

What are your early good memories of your loved one?

WAYS TO COPE

Draw or doddle something that makes you happy.

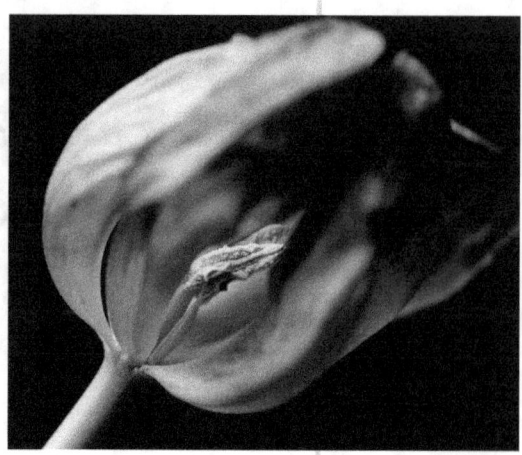

The Diagnosis

During our earlier experience with dementia, I took my mom for a doctor's visit to get some understanding of what was going on with her. She had intermittent black outs and would not remember anything before the "episode". She became extremely irritable over small things, especially with my dad who was 88. After a series of test, the doctor told me she was diagnosed with vascular dementia at age 90. I stood frozen, my heart sinking as the doctor's words echoed in my mind. The devastating news of my mother's dementia diagnosis engulfed me in a whirlwind of emotions. I did not have a clue what to expect. I guess we were in denial because we did not do the research necessary to prepare us for the journey. We felt the medication seemed to work and she seemed ok with the exception of small personality changes, surprise!

Vascular Dementia is caused by damage to the blood vessels that supply the brain, and it often occurs after a stroke. People with vascular dementia may experience sudden changes in cognitive function, including difficulty with coordination, speech, and vision. They may also have trouble with planning and decision-making and be more prone to falls.

In the days that followed, I grappled with a mix of disbelief, fear, and an overwhelming sense of sadness. Waves of uncertainty washed over me as I tried to understand the magnitude of what lay ahead. Not only for me, but for my dad who had to live with this daily. Amidst what was going through my mind, a small quiet voice said " I am with you the entire journey. You are not alone." I have an abundance of faith and I walk my Spiritual walk daily, so I knew who was whispering in my ear. I was resolved to face this new reality head-on, ready to navigate the uncharted waters of caregiving with unwavering love and strength.

Slowly, over the next nine years, her behavior became more erratic, she became more forgetful, and her mood was in constant change, I was physically losing her even though she was present and that feeling, or emotion seems like an eternity, until that day she transitioned.

I began embarking on a relentless quest for knowledge. While holding down my day job, late into the night, I immersed myself in articles, books, and expert advice, absorbing every piece of information I could find about dementia. The more I learned, the better equipped I felt to provide the care my mother needed. Armed with this newfound knowledge, I still felt lost and alone in this battle. No, I did not connect with support groups or online communities because it just did not come to mind. Afterwards, I thought, "I should have" because I might not had felt alone in this. That support would have been consistent with people who were experiencing the battle WITH me versus been through it and that makes a huge difference. I was able to fight through on my Faith, close friends, and select family members.

I poured my emotions into phone texts I would send myself on early morning walks. My text/journal became a sanctuary, a private space where I could unleash the torrent of feelings swirling within me. I wrote of my love for my mother, new insights, the pain of witnessing her decline, and the uncertainty that loomed over her future. The act of putting my thoughts and emotions into words became a cathartic release, a way to validate my feelings and find a sense of clarity amidst the chaos.

As the days turned into weeks, I discovered the power of self-care. I realized that to be the pillar of support my mother needed and keep my sanity, I had to nurture myself as well. As mentioned earlier, I found solace in nature, taking long walks in the park, allowing the fresh air to rejuvenate my spirit. Through meditation and visualization, I learned to quiet the noise and the chatter in my mind and find moments of peace amidst the storm. I prayed incessantly and cried often at night. These self-care practices became my lifeline, reminding myself that I, too, deserved love and care during this trying time.

Though the pain of my mother's diagnosis remained, I began to glimpse a flicker of acceptance and resilience within herself. I understood that I couldn't change the course of my mother's illness, but I could make a profound difference in the moments we shared, especially when she had her lucid moments. I chose to focus on the present, cherishing each precious interaction, regardless of the challenges I faced. Through gentle words, a comforting touch, and a patient heart, I embarked on this journey with my mother, navigating the unpredictable terrain of dementia one step at a time.

In the midst of my emotional episodes, I found myself looking at the family photo albums that lined the bookshelves and the digital pictures taken over the years. As I delicately turned the pages, my heart swelled with both joy and sorrow. Each faded photograph captured moments of shared laughter, cherished milestones, and the unbreakable bond between a mother and daughter.

Tears streamed down my cheeks as I realized that while my mother's memories may fade, the love we shared would forever be etched in her heart. It was in these quiet moments, surrounded by the tangible remnants of our shared history, that I found strength and resilience. I held onto those precious memories like lifelines, providing me with the courage to face the challenges that lay ahead. In the face of my mother's dementia, I was determined to ensure that our story continued to be written with love, compassion, and unwavering devotion.

Moments are like

RARE JEWELS.

Would you pass by

ONE

without admiring it?

SEIZE THE MOMENT,
BE IN THE MOMENT

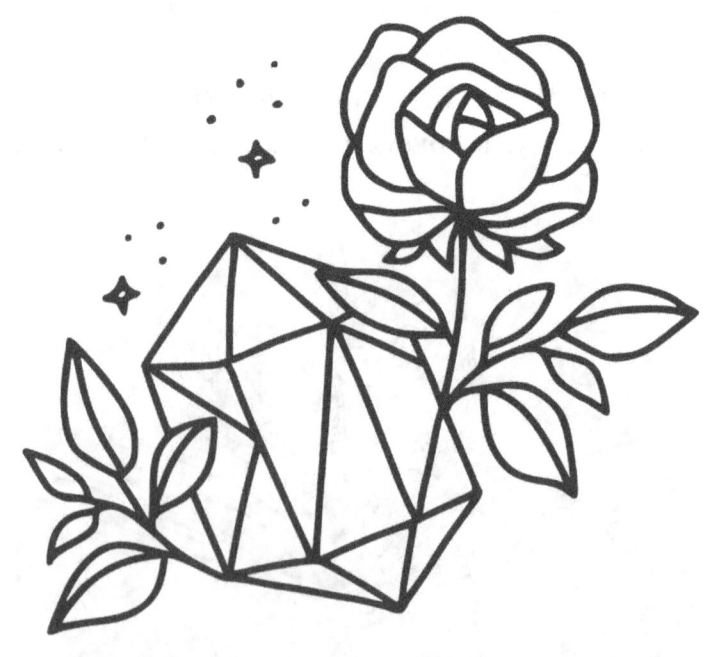

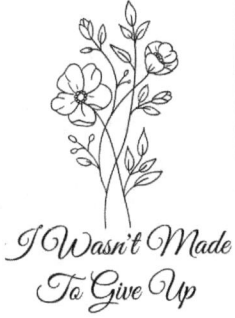

I Wasn't Made To Give Up

REFLECTIONS

What are you thinking or feeling since you learned of your loved one's dementia diagnosis?

WAYS TO COPE

TAKE A LONG WALK

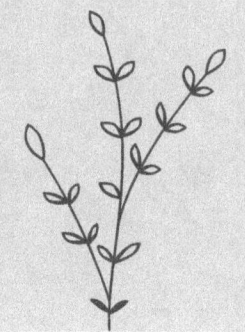

Walking is a simple yet effective coping strategy that can help you navigate the challenges of life with greater ease and clarity. Whether you're dealing with stress, anxiety, or simply need a moment of calm, taking a walk can work wonders for your physical and mental well-being.

Why walking? Walking is a natural and accessible activity that offers a multitude of benefits:

1. Stress Reduction:
Walking helps to reduce the levels of stress hormones in your body, promoting relaxation and a sense of calm
.

2. Improved Mood:
Physical activity releases endorphins, which are often referred to as "feel-good" hormones. These can boost your mood and reduce symptoms of anxiety and depression.

3. Enhanced Creativity:
Taking a walk, especially in a natural setting, can stimulate creativity and problem-solving abilities.

WAYS TO COPE

TAKE A LONG WALK

4. Increased Focus:
Regular walks can improve concentration and cognitive function, making it easier to tackle daily challenges.

5. Better Sleep:
Walking can contribute to better sleep patterns, helping you feel more rested and ready to face the day.

How to Incorporate Walking into Your Coping Routine

1. Set Aside Time:
Dedicate specific times during your day for a walk. It could be a morning stroll to start your day positively or an evening walk to unwind.

2. Choose Your Environment:
Opt for a setting that suits your mood. A peaceful park, a bustling city street, or a quiet neighborhood can all offer unique benefits.

WAYS TO COPE

TAKE A LONG WALK

3. Mindful Walking:
Use your walk as an opportunity for mindfulness. Pay attention to the sights, sounds, and sensations around you. Focus on your breath and let go of troubling thoughts.

4. Connect with Nature:
If possible, walk in a natural setting like a forest, beach, or botanical garden. Nature has a calming effect on the mind.

5. Listen to Music or Podcasts:
Bring along your favorite music or listen to an inspiring podcast to make your walk more enjoyable.

6. Walking with a Friend:
Sharing a walk with a friend or family member can provide an opportunity to talk and connect, enhancing your emotional well-being.

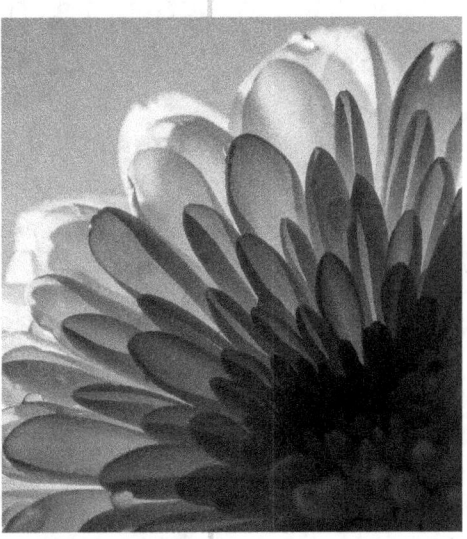

Navigating New Realities

When March 2020 rolled in, an unexpected chapter of my life began as my mother moved in with me. The world was grappling with the grip of COVID-19, and little did I know, she was also entering the final stage of her journey with dementia. At the time, she exhibited an admirable degree of independence. She managed her personal care routine, diligently prepared breakfast, and even engaged in household tasks like dishwashing, laundry, and tidying up. The quaint sight of her seated on a chair, watering the grass, became an endearing picture of her desire to contribute, even in the simplest of ways. Conversations flowed naturally, and her mood swings were, for the most part, manageable. Working remotely facilitated my role as a caregiver, allowing me to attend to her needs with relative ease. Yet, as life continued, a year would bring forth remarkable changes, shaping the course of our days in ways we could never have imagined.

By September 2020, as her 98th birthday arrived, it was becoming evident that her energy was waning. The activities that once marked her days now started to slip through her grasp. The once brisk walk around the block turned into a slower stroll, often accompanied by me by her side, offering the gentle encouragement she needed. Despite these shifts, her spirit remained undaunted. A glimmer of the woman she had always been sparkled in her eyes, especially when her great-grandchildren visited, and her 98th birthday celebration brought unparalleled delight. Sitting regally in her designated chair, she greeted guests and family as if she were the queen of the moment. However, the hours she spent at the breakfast table, gazing out the window, told stories of unspoken longing and fleeting memories.

In the arena of conversation, her fervor for politics was still palpable, though perhaps a touch less fervent than six months prior. Yet, a subtle undercurrent of change was undeniable, even if I hesitated to fully acknowledge it. The dynamic of our relationship had shifted, but my attachment to her presence and my own yearning for this novel mother-daughter companionship clouded my perception. The experience was novel, enchanting in its own way, and it was all too easy to resist acknowledging the looming shadow of what lay ahead.

The initial months of 2021 unveiled a mixture of enchantment and trepidation. During this period, my mother was still able to accompany us on travels and even venture out to the movies. Yet, there were unsettling moments that punctuated this enchantment. Episodes emerged when she began referring to my husband and me as her departed sister and brother-in-law. These moments of confusion were unsettling, jarring reminders of the gradual erosion taking place within her mind. Nights ceased to be times of restful reprieve as her sundowning behaviors emerged. She would remain awake, her agitation reflecting the turbulence of her thoughts, which meant that I, too, remained awake, tending to her needs. This nocturnal routine began to seep into my work life, forcing me to craft innovative strategies for juggling my responsibilities. Fatigue settled into my bones, a constant companion as I navigated the delicate balance between caring for her and maintaining my own equilibrium.

As the months got more difficult, I had the support of my husband, grown children, grandchildren, friends, and family. I also realized that everyone is not as fortunate to have a community to help them, and I was blessed.

BE STILL

Psalm 46:10

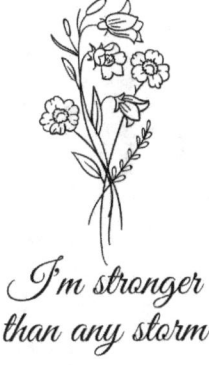

I'm stronger than any storm

REFLECTIONS

What challenges did you anticipate or face as you realized caring for your loved was going to be difficult?

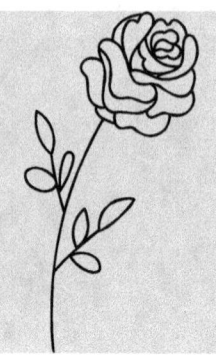

PUT YOUR TO-DO LIST ON PAUSE

Putting your to-do list on pause is a valuable coping strategy that allows you to take a break, relieve stress, and regain a sense of balance. It's essential to give yourself permission to step back from your tasks and responsibilities when needed. Here's a suggested format for this coping skill:

Step 1: Recognize the Need
Identify when you're feeling overwhelmed, stressed, or mentally fatigued. Recognizing the need for a pause is the first step in practicing this coping skill.

Step 2: Find a Quiet Space
If possible, find a quiet and comfortable space where you can sit or lie down without distractions. This could be a cozy corner, a comfortable chair, or even your bed.

Step 3: Take a Deep Breath
Before you begin, take a few deep breaths to calm your mind. Inhale deeply through your nose, hold your breath for a few seconds, and then exhale slowly through your mouth. Repeat this a few times to help you relax.

Put Your To-Do List on PAUSE

Step 4: Make a Conscious Decision
Decide to put your to-do list on pause intentionally. Understand that taking a break is a necessary part of self-care and maintaining your mental well-being.

Step 5: Set a Time Limit
Determine how long you'd like your pause to last. It could be a short break of 15-30 minutes or a more extended period, like an hour or two. Setting a time limit helps you balance your need for rest with your responsibilities.

Step 6: Disconnect from Tasks
During your pause, consciously disconnect from your to-do list and any ongoing tasks. This means stepping away from work, household chores, or any other responsibilities that can wait.

Step 7: Engage in Relaxing Activities
Choose activities that help you relax and rejuvenate. Here are some ideas:

- Deep Breathing: Practice deep breathing exercises to reduce stress and anxiety.

PUT YOUR TO-DO LIST ON PAUSE

- Meditation: Spend a few moments in meditation to clear your mind.
- Listen to Music: Play soothing or uplifting music that you enjoy.
- Read: Dive into a book, magazine, or article that brings you pleasure.
- Go for a Walk: Take a leisurely stroll outdoors to connect with nature.
- Stretching or Yoga: Engage in gentle stretching or yoga to release tension.
- Mindful Eating: Savor a snack or meal mindfully, paying attention to flavors and textures.

Step 8: No Guilt Allowed
Remind yourself that it's okay to take this break. There's no need to feel guilty about putting your to-do list on hold. Self-care is essential for maintaining your overall well-being.

Step 9: Return Refreshed
After your pause, return to your to-do list with a refreshed mindset. You'll likely find that a brief break has helped you regain focus and energy, making you more effective in your tasks.

Put Your To-Do List on PAUSE

Step 10: Repeat as Needed

Remember that putting your to-do list on pause can be a regular practice. Whenever you feel overwhelmed or stressed, don't hesitate to take another break. It's a simple but effective way to care for your mental and emotional health.

Putting your to-do list on pause is a self-compassionate act that allows you to recharge and reset. It's a reminder that your well-being is a priority, and by taking breaks when needed, you can approach your tasks and responsibilities with greater clarity and resilience.

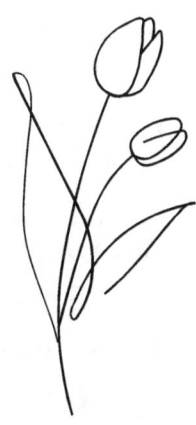

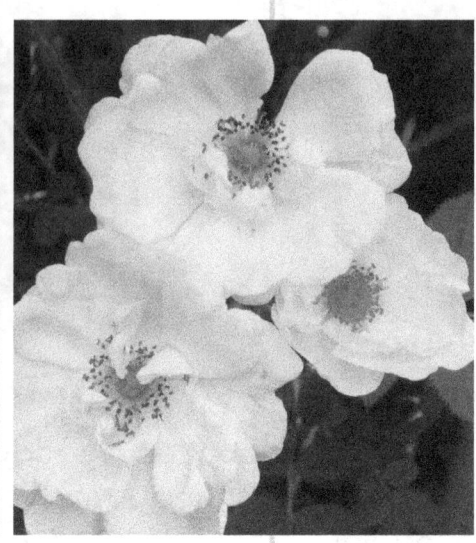

Moments of Connection

Amid the winding journey through the journey of dementia, my mother and I forged connections that felt like whispers across time itself. Often, her fragmented memories would lead us back to a world untouched by the years, where she would recount tales of her family's resilience during the Depression era. As she spoke of those trying times, her voice would soften, drawing me into the past, as she spoke about how her generation worked to make a better life for their children.

One radiant afternoon, we ventured to a restaurant nestled in a distant part of the city. The moment our feet crossed the threshold, a spark ignited in my mother's eyes, and the stories began to flow like a river of recollections. She delighted me with tales of her youth, a time when she cleaned the homes of prominent figures in the very neighborhood that surrounded us. Her voice, a gentle cadence of nostalgia, wove a tapestry of lives lived with perseverance. We delved into the struggles families endured, the creative ways they pieced together livelihoods, and the profound sense of pride that emerged from the shared pursuit of a brighter future. The glimmer of her past radiated through her gaze, a testament to the generations that had toiled for the betterment of their children's lives.

Amidst the tangled threads of memory, my mother's love for playing cards remained unscathed, a constant anchor to the past. However, the decline of her memory injected a certain complexity into the simplicity of the game. During a game of her favorite, Straight Whist, a slip occurred as she reneged on a book she had made. Our challenge was met with her characteristic response, "I'm an old lady," punctuated by her trademark cackle of laughter. In that moment, the game transcended its rules, becoming a poignant reminder of her spirit, her wit, and the endearing facets of her personality that remained untouched by the passage of time.

And then, there were the family reunion pictures, a collage of faces and memories spanning generations. We gathered around them, fingers tracing the lines of familiar smiles and cherished moments. Each image held stories, anecdotes, and the echo of laughter that once filled the air. Yet, bittersweet shadows loomed as we realized how many of those beloved faces were no longer present in our lives. The years had woven a complex tapestry, and as we immersed ourselves in those snapshots frozen in time, we found solace in the echoes of love and togetherness that persisted, undaunted by the march of time.

In the tapestry of our shared experiences, moments of connection blossomed like fragile blooms, their beauty was made even more special because it didn't last forever. Through the fragments of recollections, the glint of a shared laugh, and the depths of conversation, my mother and I created a mosaic that defied the boundaries of her condition.

L
O
V
E

Love is patient,
love is kind.
It does not envy,
it does not boast,
it is not proud.
It does not dishonor others,
it is not self-seeking,
it is not easily angered,
it keeps no record of wrongs.
Love does not delight in evil
but rejoices with the truth.
It always protects,
always trusts,
always hopes,
always perseveres.

Love never fails.

1 CORINTHIANS 13:4-13

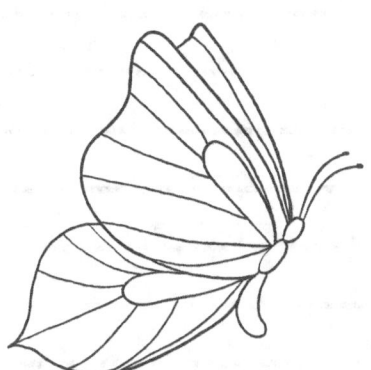

I'm Thankful For Family

REFLECTIONS

Recall you own moments of connection with loved ones and share how those moments brought you joy.

WAYS TO COPE

TAKE A DAY FOR SELF-CARE

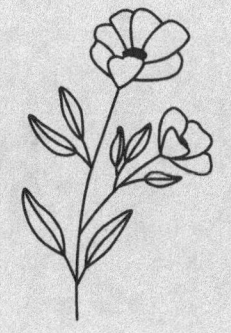

Taking a dedicated day for self-care is an essential coping strategy that allows you to recharge, rejuvenate, and prioritize your well-being. This day is all about you, and it can help reduce stress and improve your mental and emotional resilience. Here's a suggested format for this coping skill:

Step 1: Schedule Your Self-Care Day
Choose a specific day when you can dedicate time to self-care. Mark it on your calendar or set a reminder to ensure that you prioritize this day for yourself.

Step 2: Clear Your Schedule
In the days leading up to your self-care day, try to minimize commitments and responsibilities. Clear your schedule as much as possible to create a sense of freedom and relaxation.

Step 3: Plan Your Activities
Think about the activities that bring you joy, relaxation, and a sense of well-being. Plan a mix of activities that cater to your physical, emotional, and mental needs.

WAYS TO COPE

TAKE A DAY FOR SELF-CARE

Here are some ideas:

Morning:
- Start your day with a healthy breakfast.
- Engage in a calming morning meditation or yoga session.
- Spend some time journaling or reflecting on your feelings and goals.

Midday:
- Take a long, leisurely bath or shower.
- Enjoy a delicious and nourishing lunch.
- Engage in a creative activity you love, like painting, crafting, or playing a musical instrument.

Afternoon:
- Go for a nature walk or hike to connect with the outdoors.
- Practice deep breathing exercises or mindfulness to reduce stress.
- Read a book, listen to music, or watch a movie that brings you joy.

TAKE A DAY FOR SELF-CARE

Evening:
- Prepare a special, self-care dinner for yourself.
- Consider a soothing skincare routine.
- Wind down with a relaxing activity like gentle stretching or a warm cup of herbal tea.

Step 4: Disconnect from Technology

On your self-care day, minimize your use of electronic devices and social media. Unplugging from technology can help you fully immerse yourself in your chosen activities and reduce distractions.

Step 5: Prioritize Self-Care

Throughout the day, consciously prioritize your well-being. Listen to your body and mind. If you need rest, take a nap. If you're hungry, savor a nutritious meal. If you feel like dancing, put on your favorite music and dance!

Step 6: Practice Mindfulness

Stay present in the moment. Embrace each activity with mindfulness, savoring the sensations and experiences as they come. Mindfulness can help you fully enjoy your self-care day.

WAYS TO COPE

TAKE A DAY FOR SELF-CARE

Step 7: Reflect and Journal

At the end of your self-care day, take some time to reflect on how you feel. Write in a journal about your experiences, emotions, and any insights gained during the day. This reflection can help you appreciate the benefits of self-care.

Step 8: Make Self-Care a Habit

Use your self-care day as a starting point for integrating self-care into your regular routine. Consider scheduling regular moments of self-care throughout the week to maintain balance and well-being in your life.

Taking a day for self-care is a powerful way to recharge and show yourself the love and care you deserve. It's a reminder that your well-being is a priority, and it can help you better cope with the challenges and stressors of everyday life.

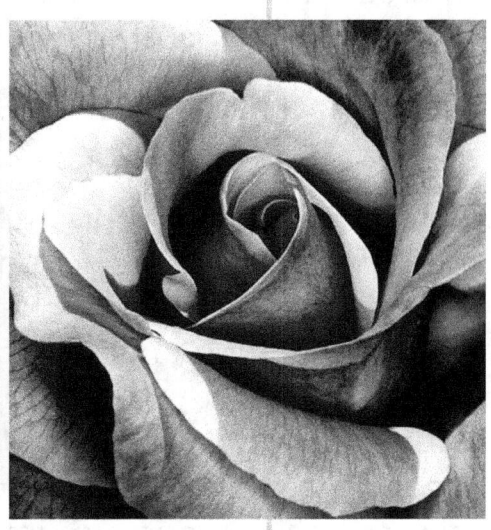

The Weight of Caregiving

Navigating the uncharted waters of caregiving was a journey I had never anticipated. My role had once been that of a parent, guiding my children and tending to the needs of my grandchildren – a different kind of responsibility. Yet, as my parents grew older and dementia settled into my mother's life, a new chapter emerged, one marked by the weight of this intricate role.

Amid the variety of my days, fatigue became an unwelcome companion, its presence magnified at the most inconvenient moments, like during my crucial work meetings. There were times when I'd be lasered focus and alert, only for the waves of exhaustion to suddenly crash over me. I recall a phase when my mother attempted to return to a place she called home for 67 years. Those nights became marathons, my granddaughter and I becoming sentinels, making sure of no escape. The memory of her peeking down the stairs, her makeshift luggage made of Walmart bags, and our shared secret still tugs at my lips, a testament to the unexpected humor that threads through even the darkest of times.

During these challenges, a sense of sadness would sometimes descend upon me, a reminder of the things that dementia had stolen. There were moments of isolation, a yearning to share my career triumphs with the mother who once stood by my side. And then there were the heart-wrenching episodes when her reality crumbled, replaced by hallucinations and moments of uncharacteristic hostility. Seeing the loving mother, I'd always known transform into a stranger, only to revert in the blink of an eye, carved a path of emotional turbulence. In those tumultuous moments, I found solace in the arms of my husband, a sanctuary of comfort and understanding. And when the weight of the journey felt unbearable, my community of Sisters became a lifeline, offering a space to share, heal, and persevere.

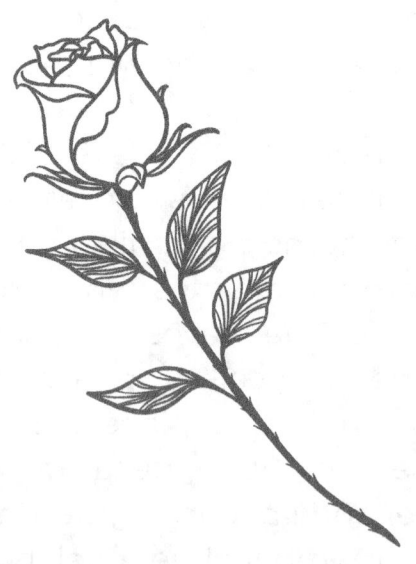

The rhythm of my personal life shifted as the tendrils of caregiving tightened their grip. Self-care, once a lifeline, slipped through the cracks. It was in this dance of adjustment that my husband and I carved new avenues for rejuvenation. Friends gathered on our deck, their laughter infusing the air with a sense of release. Inside, my grandkids watched over "Granny Turner," a testament to the beauty of connection even when the path is difficult.

Yet, amidst the chaos, some moments stung with a poignant ache. Each morning, as I struggled to rouse my mother from slumber, her words echoed like a refrain: "I'm dying." The anguish of coaxing her into the realm of the present, tugging her from the embrace of dreams, was an emotional battlefield. On days when our efforts bore fruit, there was a semblance of calm. But on the days when the struggle prevailed, frustration reigned, and I reluctantly allowed her to linger in sleep, hoping for a gentler dawn.

Even now, the mere thought of coaxing the unwilling from sleep is a trigger, stirring echoes of that challenging time. The weight of caregiving, with its myriad facets, has become a mosaic of memories, some tender, others painful, but all indelibly etched into the tapestry of my journey.

As you experience the ebb and flow of this journey, one truth stands steadfast: the significance of seeking support. As these words find their way to your eyes, it is a reminder like a guiding beacon, if you haven't already, extend your hand and let others in. The weight of caregiving is a mantle too heavy to bear alone.

Imagine your path as a road, winding through unpredictable terrains. Each curve presents new hurdles, and it's easy to lose your way. But, envision the people around you as signposts, guiding lights that illuminate the dark corners and offer solace in the face of uncertainty. They stand ready to share the burden, to lend a hand, to listen, and to understand.

In this moment, don't hesitate to reach out, for vulnerability is not a sign of weakness, but a testament to your strength. Share your experiences, your struggles, and your hopes with those willing to offer a listening ear or a comforting embrace. Whether it's a partner, a friend, a support group, or a community of individuals who have tread similar paths, remember that in forging these connections, you're forging lifelines that can provide respite from the storm.

For in the collective embrace of shared experiences, you'll find camaraderie, a space to vent the unspoken frustrations, and a source of empathy that only those who've walked a similar path can truly provide. Open your heart to their presence, for they possess the capacity to kindle a spark of strength within you, to uplift your spirit when the journey feels too arduous to bear alone.

"Stress is not what happens to us. It's our response to what happens. And response is something we can choose."

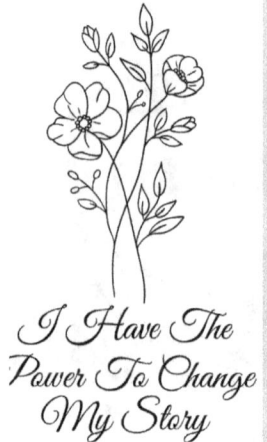

I Have The Power To Change My Story

REFLECTIONS

Evaluate your own self-care practices. Is there something you are neglecting to do for your own health and well-being?

WAYS TO COPE

PRACTICE GRATITUDE

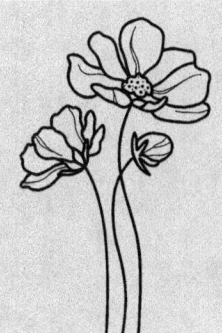

Practicing gratitude is a powerful coping strategy that can shift your focus from what is challenging in your life to what is positive and uplifting. Making a list of things you are grateful for is a simple but effective exercise that can boost your mood and overall well-being. Here is a suggested format for this coping skill:

Step 1: Find a Quiet and Comfortable Space
Begin by finding a peaceful and comfortable place where you can sit or write without distractions. It could be a cozy corner in your home, a park bench, or anywhere that allows you to relax.

Step 2: Take a Deep Breath
Before you start, take a moment to take a deep breath. Inhale slowly through your nose, hold it for a few seconds, and then exhale slowly through your mouth. This can help you center yourself and create a positive atmosphere.

Step 3: Set an Intention
Set an intention for your gratitude practice. Decide how many things you would like to list, whether it is a

Practice gratitude

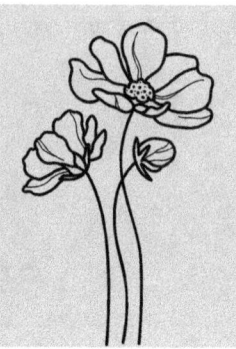

specific number or simply as many as come to mind. Setting an intention helps focus your practice.

Step 4: Start Writing
Begin writing down the things you are grateful for. These can be big or small, simple, or significant. They may include people, experiences, possessions, or aspects of your life. Write freely without overthinking it .

Step 5: Be Specific and Detailed
When listing items, try to be specific and detailed. Instead of writing "family," you might write "my supportive and loving family who always has my back." Specificity adds depth to your gratitude.

Step 6: Reflect on Each Item
As you write each item on your list, take a moment to reflect on why you are grateful for it. What positive impact has it had on your life? How does it make you feel?

Step 7: Use All Your Senses
Engage your senses when listing items. Consider things

PRACTICE GRATITUDE

you can see, hear, touch, taste, or smell that brings you joy or comfort. This multi-sensory approach enhances your gratitude practice.

Step 8: Include Yourself

Don't forget to include yourself in your list. Acknowledge your qualities, achievements, and the positive choices you've made. Self-gratitude is equally important.

Step 9: Keep Your List

Save your gratitude list in a safe and easily accessible place. You can revisit it whenever you need a mood boost or a reminder of the positive aspects of your life.

Step 10: Make It a Habit

Practice gratitude regularly. Set aside time each day or week to make new entries on your list. Cultivating this habit can help you maintain a positive outlook on life.

Practicing gratitude can shift your perspective and enhance your overall well-being. It allows you to recognize and appreciate the abundance in your life, no

WAYS TO COPE

Practice gratitude

matter how small or large. By making a list of things you are grateful for, you create a tangible record of positivity that can be a source of comfort and inspiration during challenging times.

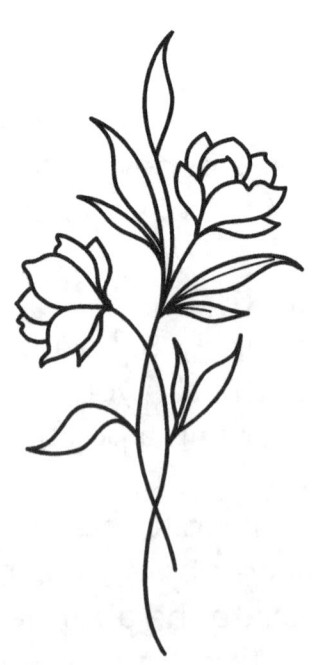

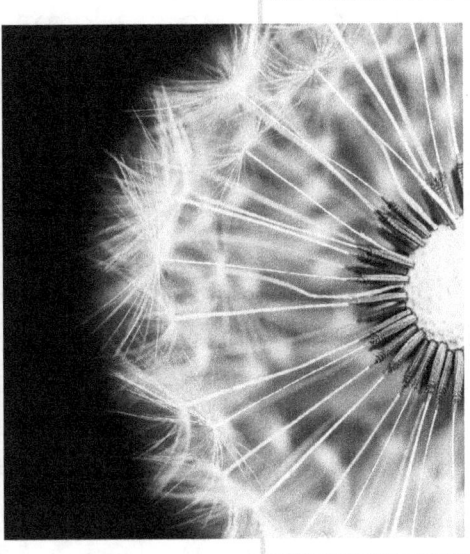

Facing the Inevitable

Labor Day Weekend of 2021 etched a chapter of profound gravity in our journey. Loyola Hospital became the stage for a confluence of elements that heralded an inevitable shift. My mother, once a bastion of strength, had become a reflection of fragility. Her blood pressure, a measure of life's vitality, surged to 200/100, while sleep remained an elusive dream for two torturous days. A haunting symphony of symptoms began to weave its melody – diminished appetite, an ominous departure from her love for indulgent desserts, and an agitation that colored her world with disarray. Hallucinations danced before her eyes, and her emotions swung like a pendulum of chaos.

Within the sterile confines of the hospital, a series of tests were conducted, a cascade of medications administered. Blood pressure was wrestled into submission, a war waged against the tormenting hallucinations, and a lullaby of tranquility coaxed her into sleep. But despite these efforts, the stark reality loomed. The once sturdy hospital bed, her sanctuary, could no longer keep her safe from the precipice of falls. A tent-like bed became her refuge, a cocoon of protection against the unpredictable hazards that lurked in her unsteady steps. The situation was stark, the most distressing I had ever witnessed. The weight of the unknown bore down on me like a storm cloud, my thoughts echoing with the chilling question: "How am I going to care for her now?"

The tension was palpable as I grappled with fear's icy grip. Then, on a day heavy with unspoken truths, the doctor entered her room. There was a hesitancy in his voice, an acknowledgement of the weight his words bore. The prognosis, unfiltered, hung between us like an unspoken vow. My mother, in her weakened state, was showing signs that whispered of the inevitable – her journey was nearing its end. A conversation that words alone cannot encompass transpired; his gaze met mine, and the unspoken agreement settled like a fragile petal on a breeze.

And so, the path was laid. Hospice Care, a gentle embrace to accompany her transition, was the decision we made. Conversations with the organization became my lifeline, a beacon guiding us through the process of creating an environment that embraced both comfort and dignity. Labor Day of 2021, a day traditionally marked by festivities, became a marker of irrevocable change. As she left the hospital's confines, the weight of reality pressed heavily upon my heart – she was no longer just battling dementia, she was now in a physical encounter with mortality itself.

In this moment, the essence of strength took on a new meaning. The landscape before us was treacherous, uncertain, yet within the uncertainty lay a grace. As the journey turned towards the inevitable, we would walk it with open hearts, embracing each step as an act of love, even as we faced the uncertainty ahead.

love between a mother and daughter is forever

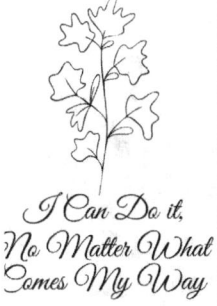

I Can Do it,
No Matter What
Comes My Way

REFLECTIONS

Contemplate the decisions you may face as a caregiver. See end-of-life care resources included in this book.

WAYS TO COPE

PRACTICE ACCEPTANCE

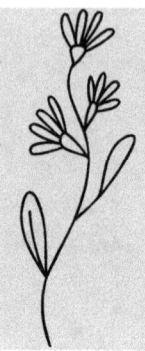

Accepting your emotions as a natural part of your experience is a valuable coping strategy. Emotions, whether positive or negative, are a normal and essential part of being human.

This practice allows you to acknowledge and embrace your feelings without judgment, ultimately helping you navigate through difficult moments. Here's a suggested format for this coping skill:

Step 1: Find a Quiet Space
To begin, find a quiet and comfortable space where you can be alone with your thoughts. This can be a calming room, a cozy corner, or any place where you feel at ease.

Step 2: Take a Deep Breath
Start by taking a deep breath. Inhale slowly through your nose, hold it for a few seconds, and then exhale slowly through your mouth. Repeat this a few times to center yourself and calm your mind.

Step 3: Acknowledge Your Emotions
Close your eyes if it helps, and bring your attention to your current emotional state. Acknowledge the

PRACTICE ACCEPTANCE

emotions you are experiencing without judgment. Whether you're feeling joy, sadness, anger, fear, or any other emotion, remember that they are all valid and natural.

Step 4: Name Your Emotions
If it helps, name the emotions you're feeling. For example, "I am feeling sadness," "I am feeling anger," or "I am feeling happiness." This can provide clarity and help you connect with your feelings.

Step 5: Observe Sensations in Your Body
Pay attention to any physical sensations associated with your emotions. Emotions often manifest as bodily sensations, such as tension, warmth, or a sinking feeling in the stomach. Observe these sensations without trying to change them.

Step 6: Remind Yourself of Impermanence
Reflect on the impermanence of emotions. Understand that emotions, like passing clouds, come and go. They are not permanent fixtures in your life, and they will eventually pass.

WAYS TO COPE

PRACTICE ACCEPTANCE

Step 7: Practice Self-Compassion
Be kind and compassionate toward yourself. It's okay to feel the way you do. Offer yourself the same understanding and care that you would offer a friend in a similar situation.

Step 8: Let Go of Judgment
Release any judgment you may have about your emotions. Avoid labeling them as "good" or "bad." Emotions simply are, and they serve as signals about what's happening in your inner world.

Step 9: Return to the Present
Open your eyes if they were closed and bring your focus back to the present moment. You've acknowledged your emotions and practiced acceptance.

Step 10: Repeat as Needed
Remember that practicing acceptance is an ongoing process. Whenever you find yourself struggling with your emotions, return to this practice to help you navigate them with greater ease and self-compassion.

WAYS TO COPE

PRACTICE ACCEPTANCE

This coping skill encourages you to embrace the full spectrum of human emotions, recognizing that they are all part of your unique experience. By accepting your emotions without judgment, you can find greater peace and resilience in the face of life's challenges.

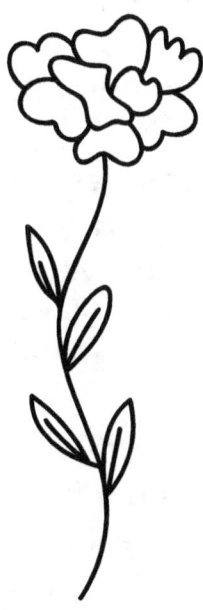

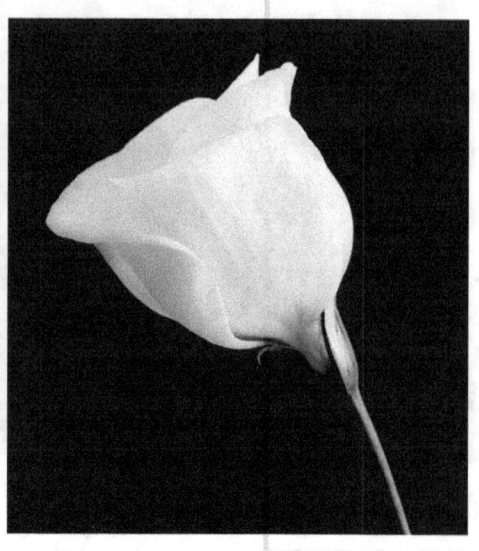

Embracing the Farewell

Throughout the stages of my life, I had always worn the mantle of a "strong woman" with faith as my guardian. It had seen me through the profound depths of hospice experiences, not once, but three times within the span of four years. So, when the moment came for what I believed would be the ultimate farewell – the "last goodbye" to my mother – I held onto the threads of my conviction. Yet, as life often unfolds, it surprised me.

Dementia, a thief of memories and a distorting mirror, wove its intricate web around my mother's thoughts. In its grip, she was led to believe that the bonds of love between us were frayed, torn. Her words carried the echo of this distorted belief, phrases like "You know I love you," laced with the poignant ache of uncertainty. My responses were whispered affirmations, a lifeline of truth, "Of course I know, you are my mom." On some days, her voice would tremble as she asked the question that held a universe of reassurance, "Do you love me?" My response was a reservoir of emotion, "More than you know," the words flowing like a river, a testament to the depth of my feelings.

In those moments, my heart ached to guide her back through the maze of her memories, to gather the fragments of shared love and weave them into her present. And then, a glimmer of clarity pierced through the fog. On her 99th birthday, surrounded by the laughter of her grandchildren, the innocent joy of great-grandchildren, the strength of her son-in-law, and the unwavering love of her daughter, she was granted a moment of lucidity. As the room filled with the melody of "Happy Birthday," her voice joined in, a proclamation of triumph, "I made it!" In that instant, we glimpsed the traces of her real self, untouched by the haze of dementia.

But it was her final moments that etched a tapestry of closure and love. A communion of hearts, an exchange of emotions unmarred by confusion. Her voice, fragile yet resolute, carried the weight of a lifetime's affection, "I love you, and we are going to be okay." My response, a whispered pledge, "I love you back, and yes, we will." In the symphony of those words, our souls intertwined one last time. With her final breath, the curtains closed on her journey, leaving behind the echoes of a love that transcended the constraints of memory.

The importance of closure, I realized, held the power to reshape the landscape of grieving. Closure was not a mere formality, but a journey unto itself. It meant mending old wounds, turning doubts into affirmations, and finally voicing what should have been said long ago. It meant standing on the precipice of goodbye with no lingering regrets, a foundation upon which grief could find its release. In the quiet aftermath, the knowledge that we had no lingering regrets became my balm, a comfort that embraced me as I navigated the stormy waters of loss.

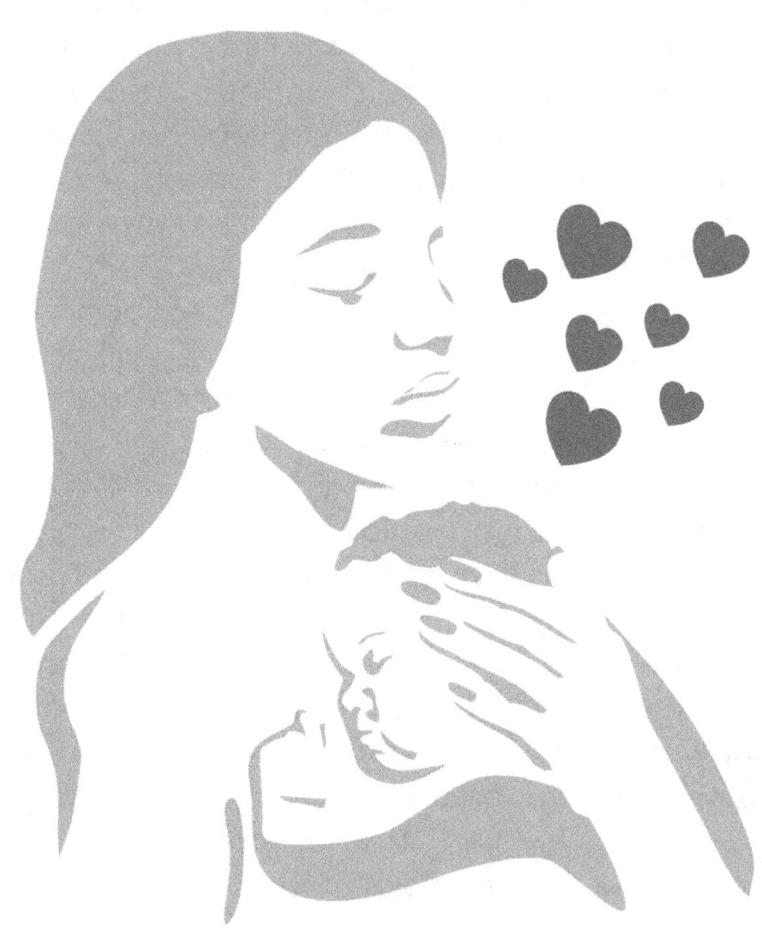

" I look at hospice as Grace...
It gave me a chance to experience my mother leaving this world as she experienced me coming into this world."

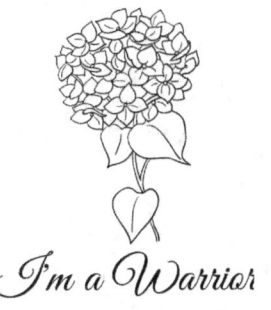

I'm a Warrior

REFLECTIONS

Reflect on your own experiences of loss and healing.

_____

_____

_____

_____

_____

_____

_____

_____

_____

_____

_____

_____

_____

_____

_____

_____

_____

_____

WAYS TO COPE

WRITE A LETTER TO YOUR LOVED ONE

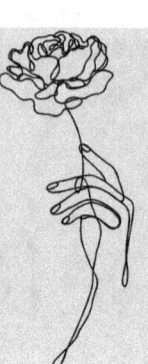

Writing a heartfelt letter to a loved one can be a therapeutic and healing coping strategy. This exercise provides a safe space for you to express your thoughts, emotions, and feelings, even if you don't plan to send the letter. It can be a powerful way to process your experiences and find closure or release pent-up emotions. Here's a suggested format for this coping skill:

Step 1: Choose a Comfortable Environment
Find a quiet and comfortable place where you can concentrate and feel at ease. This could be your favorite chair, a cozy corner of your room, or even a serene outdoor spot.

Step 2: Address Your Loved One
Start the letter by addressing your loved one by name or in a way that feels personal to you. For example, "Dear [Name]," or simply "My Dearest," depending on your relationship.

Step 3: Express Your Feelings
This is where you can let your emotions flow freely.

WRITE A LETTER TO YOUR LOVED ONE

Share your thoughts, feelings, and experiences honestly and without reservation. Describe what you're going through, what you miss about them, or any unresolved issues you want to address. This is your opportunity to communicate everything you wish you could say in person.

Step 4: Reflect and Remember
Take some time to reflect on the positive memories and moments you've shared. Recall the special times, anecdotes, and experiences that have shaped your relationship. Celebrate the love and connection you've had.

Step 5: Address Unfinished Business (Optional)
If there are unresolved issues or regrets, you may choose to address them in this letter. This can be a way to find closure or forgiveness, even if it's just for your own peace of mind.

Step 6: Share Your Hopes and Wishes
Express your hopes and wishes for your loved one, even if they can't directly hear them. This can be a way to send positive energy or healing thoughts to them, wherever they may be.

WRITE A LETTER TO
YOUR LOVED ONE

Step 7: Offer Forgiveness and Gratitude (Optional)
If applicable, consider forgiving any hurt or pain you may have experienced and express gratitude for the positive aspects of your relationship. Forgiveness and gratitude can be powerful sources of healing.

Step 8: Sign the Letter
Close the letter with a warm and loving sign-off. You might use phrases like "With all my love," "Forever in my heart," or "Yours always."

Step 9: Keep or Disposal
You have the choice to keep the letter in a safe place as a personal memento or perform a symbolic act of letting go, such as tearing it up or burning it, to symbolize release and closure.

Remember, this letter is for your personal healing and reflection. You can revisit it whenever you need to process your emotions or find solace in your memories. It can be a valuable tool for coping with the complexities of your feelings toward your loved one, whether they are with you or not.

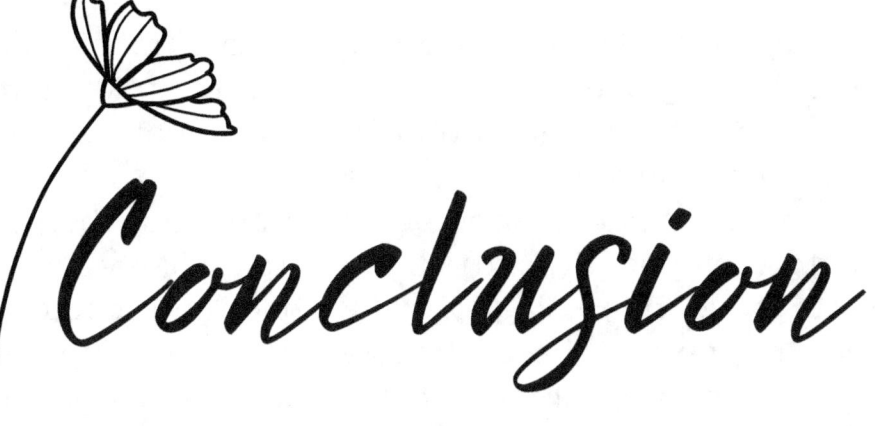

Conclusion

The Odyssey of Dementia:
An Embodiment of Life's Lessons

Dementia is a demanding and taxing journey, yet the wisdom I've gained along the way is invaluable. I've learned to cherish the present, finding solace in life's smaller joys. It's essential not to let the perpetual "busy" of life deter us from engaging with our loved ones. Time waits for no one, and the moments we share with those we hold dear are fleeting. In today's digital age, we have a remarkable tool at our disposal – recording videos of our loved ones. Personally, I've found solace in capturing my mother's voice, as playing back those videos brings a sense of lightness to my heart. Nevertheless, a word of caution – technology can be fickle, and relying solely on voicemails may prove risky.

Preserve your family's narrative by delving into its history alongside your loved ones. Uncover tales of their childhoods, trace the intricate threads of extended families, and unveil the lineage that shapes you. For when they depart, these stories often depart with them, slipping away like whispers in the wind. Embrace the significance of legacy, for it's in these stories that your roots and essence find their place in the world.

Within my journey, the concept of self-care transformed into something deeply personal – a mantra of "My Care." I embraced it with intention, realizing that to be a beacon for others, I must first tend to my own flame. Amid the ebb and flow, there were moments when the undertow of negativity threatened to pull me under. Doubts of a looming diagnosis like a haunting specter. In a bid to prevent these shadows from growing into formidable demons, I took decisive action. I sought the guidance of therapy, a lifeline to navigate the labyrinth of my thoughts and emotions. It's a step I encourage all of us on this journey to consider, for within the folds of mental health and well-being lies the strength to weather even the stormiest seas.

Lastly, as these words find their way to you, I extend a heartfelt plea: practice kindness towards yourself. It's a compass that guides you through the intricate landscapes of caregiving and living with dementia. Embrace the power of seeking understanding, for it fosters connections that transcend the barriers of this challenging journey. Let empathy be the glue that binds hearts, a bridge connecting the realms of caregivers and those touched by dementia. And remember, support is not a sign of vulnerability, but a beacon of strength. Reach out, extend a hand or lend an ear – because in these acts of compassion, we find the resilience to traverse the untrodden paths together.

RESOURCES

The Seven Stages Of Dementia
https://www.dementiasociety.org

Downloadable Resources | Alzheimer's
Association

Alzheimer's and Related Dementias
Resources for Professionals | National
Institute on Aging (nih.gov

End With Care | A Resource for End-of-Life
Care

Providing Care and Comfort at the End of
Life | National Institute on Aging (nih.gov)

The Types of Dementia Explained - United
Methodist Communities
(umcommunities.org

Tips for Caregivers and Families of People
With Dementia (alzheimers.gov

In Loving Memory of Nancy Turner

A phenomenal warrior, daughter, sister, wife, mother,
grandmother, aunt, friend, cousin, and child of God.

SEPTEMBER 22, 1922 - SEPTEMBER 24, 2021

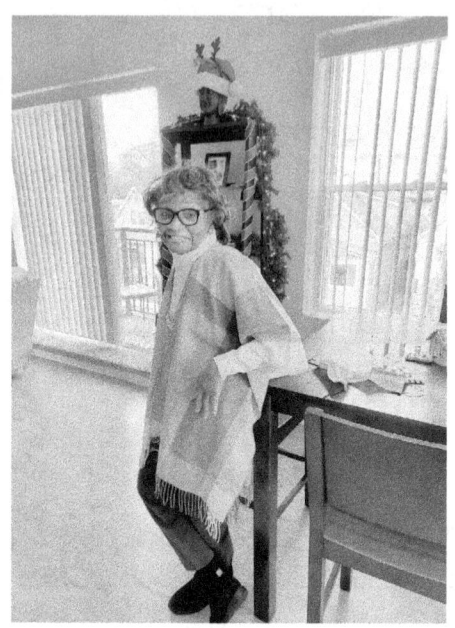
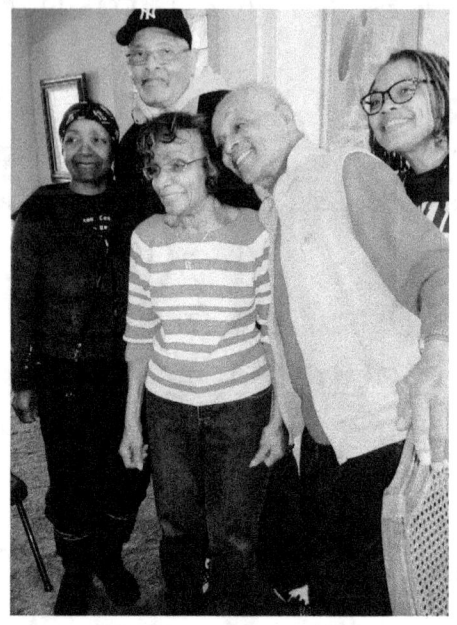

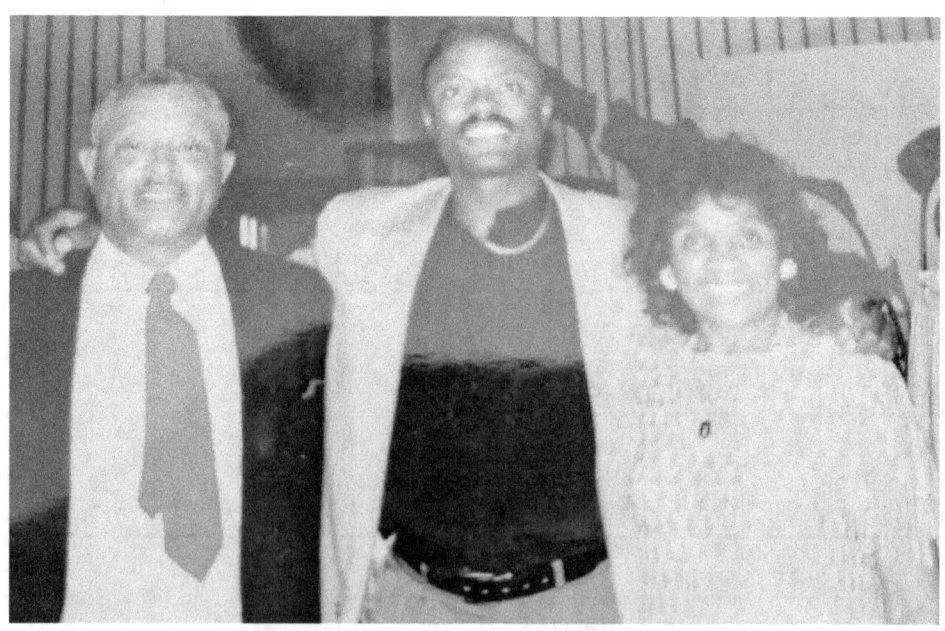

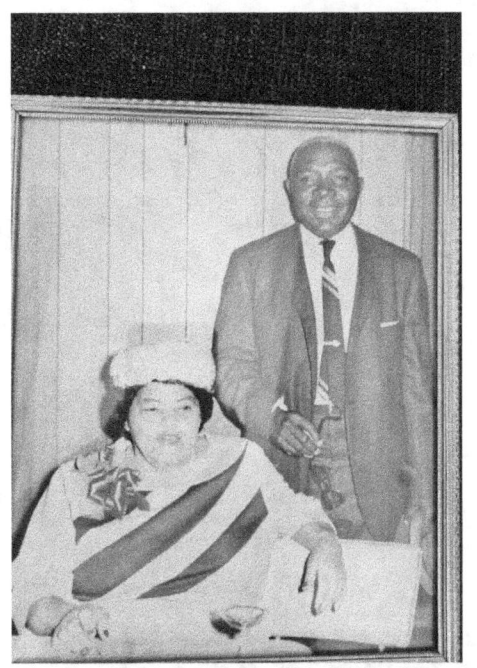

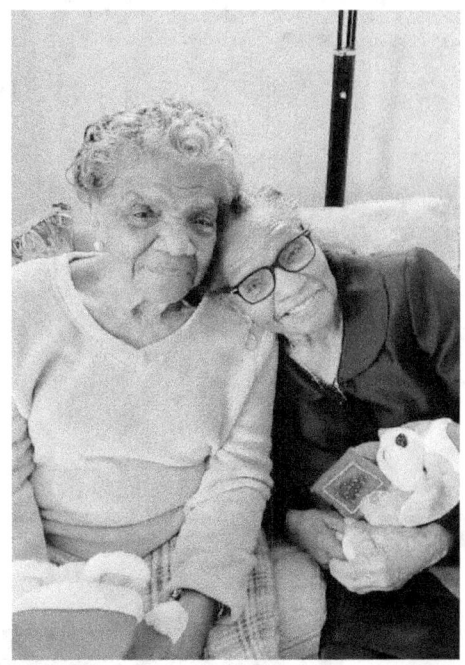

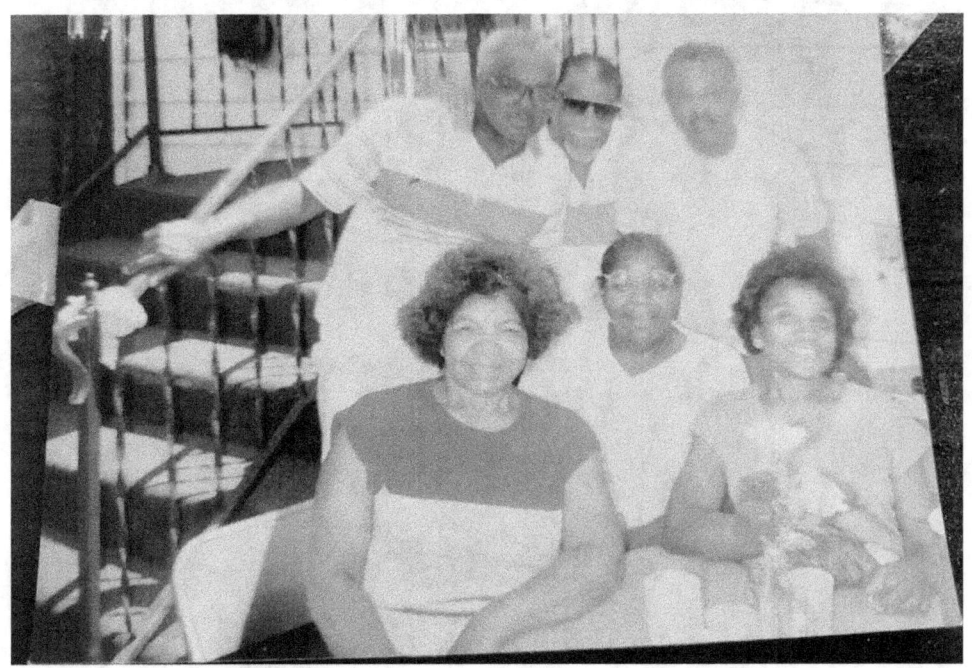

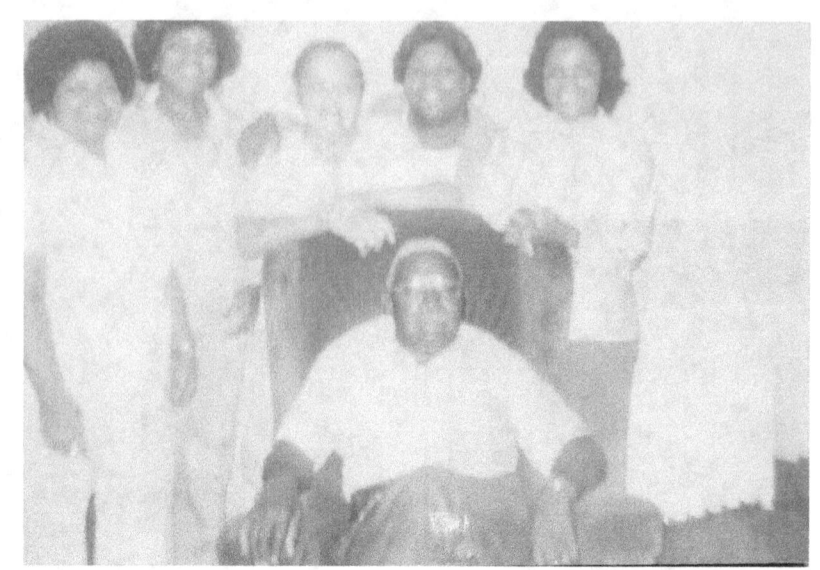

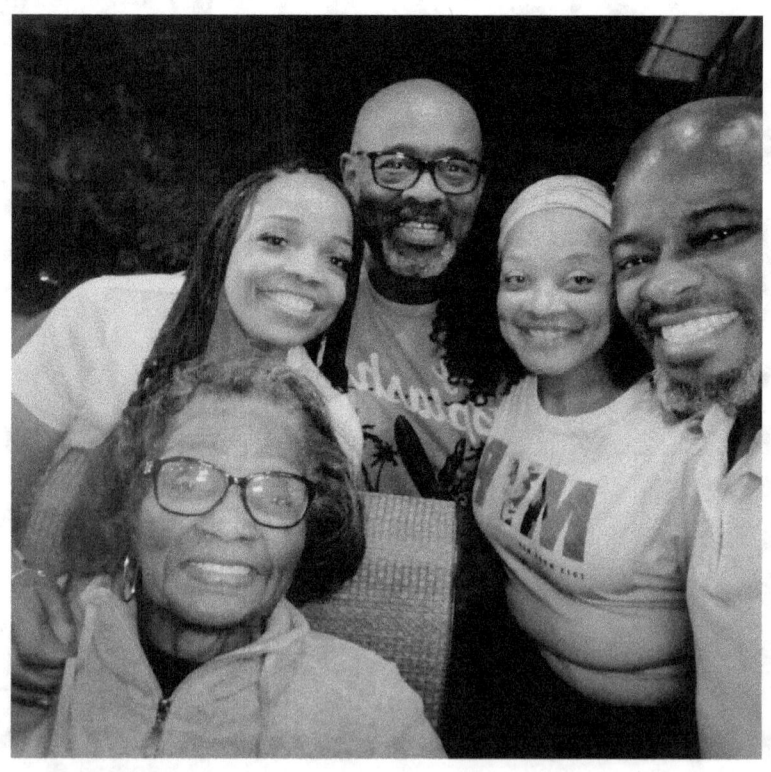

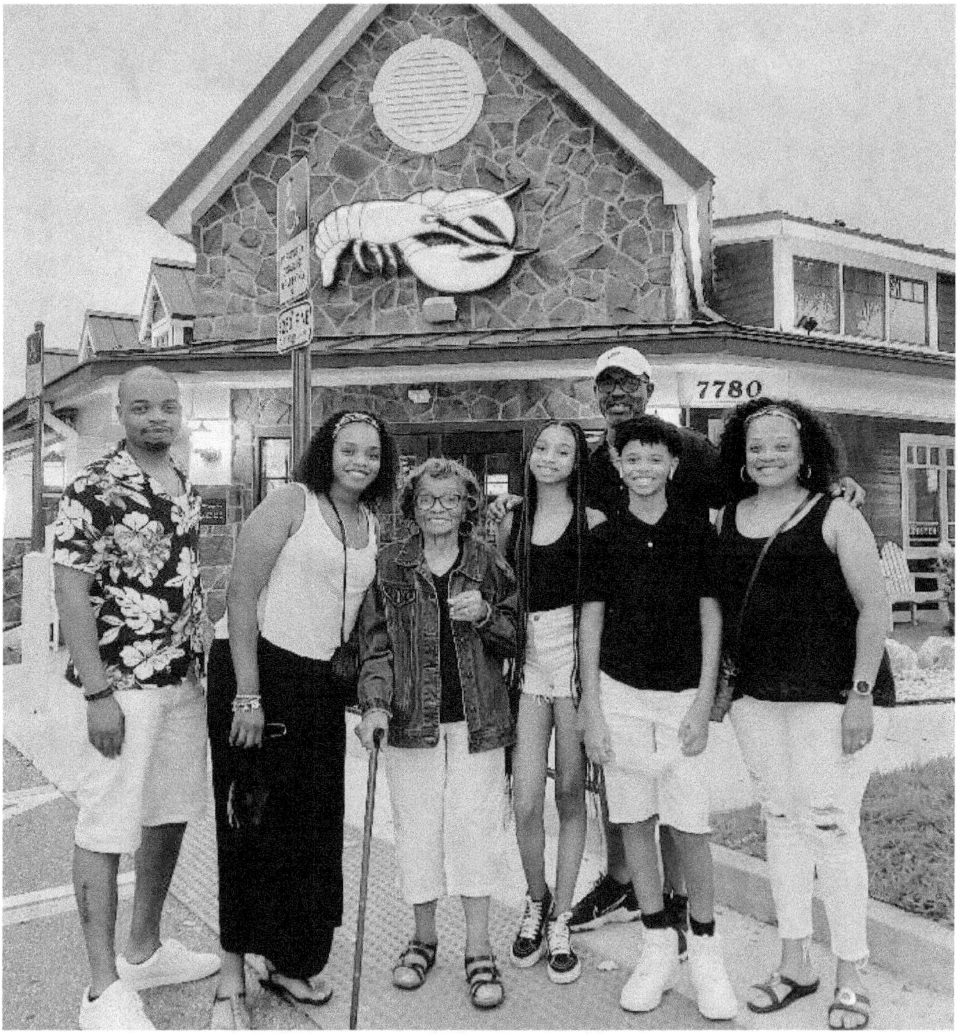

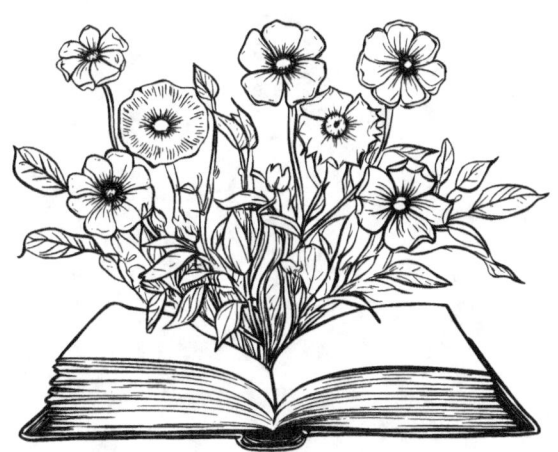

www.ingramcontent.com/pod-product-compliance
Lightning Source LLC
Chambersburg PA
CBHW062244290526
45794CB00006B/2394

* 9 7 9 8 8 6 3 6 2 9 7 7 3 *